The Migraine Diet Cookbook

Over 50 Recipes Without Common Triggers Or Additives

Help Eliminate Or Reduce The Severity And Frequency Of Migraine Attacks

Common Ingredient Substitutes

By Michelle Strong

ISBN-13: 978-1530093830
ISBN-10: 153009383X

DISCLAIMER

Disclaimer and Terms of Use: Every effort has been made to ensure that the information in this book is accurate and complete, however, the author and the publisher do not warrant the accuracy of the information and text contained within the book due to the rapidly changing nature of science, research, known and unknown facts and internet. The Author and the publisher do not hold any responsibility for errors, omissions or contrary interpretation of the subject matter herein. This book is presented solely for motivational and informational purposes only. Consult your doctor before going on any diet or exercise plan. It is best to have an effective plan on how to manage your migraines established with your doctor.

CONTENTS

INTRODUCTION

The *Migraine Diet Cookbook* is specifically for migraine sufferers who know that certain common foods and additives will trigger their migraines, either in isolation or in combination with other foods and additives, or other triggers. Other triggers can be an event, physical act, change, or external stimulus (such as weather, perfume, flickering lighting etc).

There is no cure for migraines, there can only be attempts at reducing their frequency and intensity. Prophylactic treatments can include a combination of measures such as avoiding triggers, taking prescribed medications, physical therapies, treatments such as botox, and behavioural therapies, such as relaxation and biofeedback. Abortive medications to stop a migraine once it has begun include prescription medications, and over-the-counter pain relievers. These treatments help some sufferers, but do not work for the majority, and can have side effects that are too severe for a lot of sufferers.

Identifying triggers is not always easy. The list can be long, confusing, and seems like it is never finished. The trigger occurs from either a short time before the attack or up to 6 to 8 hours. To clearly identify food triggers it is recommended to keep a diet diary. It should list all foods and amounts eaten every day, and the approximate times. The appearance of any symptoms should be noted.

When food triggers are identified, avoiding them as far as possible is advised. Eat regular, well-balanced meals, made from fresh ingredients, avoiding processed and packaged foods. Don't skip meals as fluctuating blood sugar levels are a migraine trigger.

The recipes in this book do not contain any of the common food triggers. They do contain ingredients that have nutrients that are known to be beneficial for migraine sufferers. Some of the common ingredient substitutes makes finished dishes taste even better than if they had been made with regular products.

FOODS THAT ARE GUARANTEED SAFE

The following foods are virtually guaranteed to be pain safe. They will not trigger a migraine or contribute to any other medical condition. They are:

- Rice, in particular brown rice
- Cooked orange vegetables, such as sweet potatoes or carrots
- Cooked yellow vegetables, such as summer squash
- Cooked green vegetables such as spinach, broccoli, swiss chard, celery or collards
- Fresh or cooked non-citrus fruits such as cherries, cranberries, pears, green apples
- Water: Plain or carbonated are fine.
- Condiments: small amounts of salt, vanilla extract and maple syrup

COMMON FOOD TRIGGERS

CAFFEINE
Coffee*, tea, cola, chocolate

CHOCOLATE
All kinds

MONOSODIUM GLUTAMATE (MSG)
Soups and stock cubes
Croutons and bread crumbs
Seasoned salt
Flavoured salty snacks
Gravies
Cheap buffets
Ready to eat meals
Veggie burgers
Processed meats
Processed foods
Canned foods
Chinese and other restaurant food
Check *natural flavouring* on canned foods

PROCESSED MEAT AND FISH
Canned, aged, cured, marinated, fermented, tenderized, smoked or preserved with nitrites or nitrates.
Bacon, hot dogs, salami, sausages, pepperoni, liverwurst, bologna, lunch meats, beef jerky, pates, caviar, anchovies, smoked and pickled fish,.
Avoid beef and chicken liver which are high in Tyramine

CHEESE AND OTHER DAIRY PRODUCTS
The older, more aged the cheese, the worse

Steer clear of food containing cheese
Avoid all dairy, including all milks, sour cream, yogurt, and buttermilk.

NUTS
All nuts and nut butters
Peanuts (legumes) should also be avoided

ALCOHOL AND VINEGAR
Champagne, red wine, dark heavy spirits
Condiments high in vinegar, such as ketchup, mayonnaise and mustard

FRUITS AND JUICES
Citrus fruits and their juices
Bananas – ripe
Dried fruits
Raspberries, papayas, red plums, passionfruit, dates, figs and avocados
Any fruit that is over ripe (it will be high in tyramine)

VEGETABLES
Onions
Pea pods
Sauerkraut
Beans: broad, lima, Italian, navy, fava, and lentils

FRESH BAKED GOODS CONTAINING YEAST
Less than one day old baked breads, particularly sourdough, pizza dough, bagels, soft pretzels, doughnuts, and coffee cake.

OTHER
Soy sauce
Worcestershire sauce
Liquorice

CHECK LABELS ON EVERYTHING!

*Coffee is somewhat of a conundrum; it helps some sufferers, especially when taking painkillers, but causes migraines in others.

A list of common food substitutes is provided at the end of this book.

RECIPES

STOCKS & CONDIMENTS

CHICKEN STOCK

Chicken stock/bone broth is a highly nourishing food and is easy and cheap to make. You'll be surprised at the difference in taste when you use homemade stock in your recipes. It is also delicious to drink on its own.

Total Time: 2 Hours 30 Minutes
Prep Time: 30 Minutes
Cook Time: 2 hours
Yields: 6-8 cups

Ingredients:

1-3 chicken carcasses or 3lbs (1.5 kg) chicken bones*
1½ tbsp. onion flakes or other onion substitute
2 carrots, unpeeled and roughly chopped
2 stalks celery, roughly chopped
6 parsley sprigs
1 sprig thyme
1/2 tsp. black peppercorns
2 bay leaves

Directions:

1. Place everything in a stock pot and cover with 4 inches of cold water. Bring to the boil, then lower the heat and simmer gently, uncovered for 2 or more hours. Be careful the stock does not boil too rapidly as it will become cloudy. You can also cook this in the slow cooker for 24 hours on low.
2. Let the stock cool before straining the solids into a large bowl through a sieve. The bones can be used again for another batch of stock.
3. Leave the stock settle in the fridge overnight for the fat to solidify on top. Skim it off before storing.
4. Stock can be stored in the freezer for up to 8 weeks. If freezing in glass jars leave enough room for the liquid to expand so the jars don't break.

*You can also use a whole chicken and pull the meat off the bone for use in other dishes, before straining the broth through a sieve.

Nutritional Information per serving: (Serving size: 1 cup):

Calories: 86
Fat: 2.9g
Carbs: trace
Dietary fibre: 0g
Protein: 6g
Cholesterol: 0
Sodium: 343mg

CHICKEN FEET STOCK

Total Time: 6 Hours 35 Minutes
Prep Time: 30 Minutes
Cook Time: 6 Hours 5 minutes
Yields: 8 cups

Ingredients:

2 lbs/1kg of chicken feet
2 large carrots, cut in half
1½ tbsps onion flakes or other onion substitute
2 celery stalks, cut in half
1 bunch of fresh thyme
1 bay leaf
10 peppercorns
Cheesecloth, muslin or fine mesh strainer for straining

Directions:

1. Bring 8 cups of water to the boil in a large stock pot. Add the chicken feet and boil for 5 minutes, skimming off any scum that rises to the surface with a large metal spoon.
2. Drain the chicken feet and rinse with cold water so that they are cool enough to handle. With a sharp knife or kitchen shears, cut off the tips of the claws through the first knuckle and discard. Cut away any remaining rough patches of claw pad with a paring knife.

3. Clean the stock pot and place the chicken feet back in. Fill with cold water to an inch above the chicken feet. Add all the other ingredients: onion, carrots, celery, bay leaf, thyme, and peppercorns. Bring to a simmer, then immediately reduce the temperature to low. Cover, leaving partly uncovered by about half an inch. The stock needs to cook for 4 hours at the mildest simmer. Skim off any foam that comes to the surface.
4. Uncover and increase the heat slightly, although it must still be a low simmer. Continue to simmer for another hour or two. This stage is for reducing the stock. Strain the stock well, using several layers of cheesecloth / muslin / chux or a fine mesh strainer, or optimally both. Allow to cool before storing in the refrigerator overnight and skimming off the fat the next day.

Store in the freezer in plastic containers.

Nutritional Information per serving: (Serving size: 1 cup):

Calories: 60
Fat: 4g
Carbs: 0
Dietary fibre: 0
Protein: 5g
Cholesterol: 24mg
Sodium: 19mg

BEEF STOCK

Total Time: 6 Hours
Prep Time: 1 Hour 15 Minutes
Cook Time: 4 Hours 45 Minutes
Yields: 10 cups

Ingredients:

3 lbs (1.5kg) beef bones
1½ tbsps onion flakes or other onion substitute
2 carrots, unpeeled and roughly chopped
2 stalks celery, halved
6 sage leaves
1 sprig of thyme
1 sprig of rosemary
2 bay leaves
2 sprigs flat-leaf parsley
salt and pepper to taste
Cheesecloth, muslin or fine mesh strainer for straining

Directions:

Preheat oven to 445°F/230°C.
1. Roast beef bones and vegetables for 1 hour 30 minutes, turning occasionally, or until browned.
2. Fill a large stock pot with 1.3 gallons5 (litres) cold water and add the roasted beef bones and vegetables, scraping the roasting pan.
3. Add the bay leaves, herbs, salt and pepper.
4. Over medium high bring the stock to a boil, then lower heat and simmer for 3 or more hours.
5. Skim off any fat that rises to the top with a metal spoon.

6. Let the pot and contents cool.
7. For a clear broth, strain through cheesecloth, muslin or a chux and a metal strainer.
8. Refrigerate it and skim off the fat.

Refrigerate for up to 3 days.
Freeze up to 3 months.

Nutritional Information per serving: (Serving size: 1 cup):

Calories: 31
Fat: 0g
Carbs: 3g
Dietary fibre: 0g
Protein: 5.2g
Cholesterol: 0mg
Sodium: 475mg

VEGETABLE STOCK

Total Time: 1 Hour
Prep Time: 10 Minutes
Cook Time: 50 Minutes
Yields: 4/5 cups

Ingredients:

1½ tbsps onion flakes or other onion substitute
2 carrots, roughly chopped into big chunks
2 stalks celery, roughly chopped into big chunks
1 leek, top green leaves only, roughly chopped
2 cloves of garlic, smashed
salt and pepper to taste
4 sprigs parsley
1 bay leave
4 sprigs thyme
6 cups cold water
Cheesecloth, muslin or fine mesh strainer

Directions:

1. Tie the bay leaf, parsley and thyme together with kitchen string.
2. Place all the ingredients into an 8 quart (8 litre) stockpot. Use a medium heat to bring to the boil, and then reduce to low and simmer for approx. 30 minutes, until liquid has loads of flavour.
3. Remove from heat. Strain into a large bowl/pot through a fine sieve lined with muslin / cheesecloth / chux cloth. Discard solids. Simmer stock to reduce and intensify flavour, if needed.

4. Let cool. Keep refrigerated for up to 4 days or freeze for up to 3 months.

Nutritional Information per serving: (Serving size: 1 cup):

Calories: 12
Fat: 0g
Carbs: 3g
Dietary fibre: 2g
Protein: 0g
Cholesterol: 0mg
Sodium: 940mg

THAI CURRY PASTE

Total Time: 25 Minutes
Prep Time: 25 Minutes

Ingredients:

1 head of garlic, peeled
2 stalks lemongrass, thinly sliced
2 inches fresh galangal, sliced
The peel of 1 kaffir lime, sliced, or 10 fresh kaffir lime leaves, middle stem removed and thinly sliced
1/2 tsp. salt
15 whole dried chillies
1 tbsp shrimp paste/sauce (read the label to ensure you are only getting shrimp and salt in the jar)

Directions:

Using a mortar and pestle, add ingredients in this order, pounding until each ingredient is pulverised:

1. Garlic
2. Lemongrass
3. Galangal
4. Kaffir lime peel/leaves
5. Salt
6. Whole dried chillies (it should be paste-like now)

7. Shrimp paste (read the label to ensure you are only getting shrimp and salt in the jar)

This is the basis of a very good ready to use red curry paste. To enrich the flavour, add roasted coriander seeds, roasted cumin seeds, whole white peppercorns, fresh coriander root, and shallots.

Nutritional Info per serving:

Calories: 25
Fat: 1.5g
Carbs: 2g
Dietary fibre: 1g
Protein: 2.2g
Sodium: 2656mg
Cholesterol: 50mg

Green Curry Paste:

Use the basic recipe, substituting fresh green chillies instead of whole dried chillies. Adjust the flavours as indicated above.

THAI FRIED SHALLOTS

Total Time: 5 Minutes
Prep Time: 3 Minutes
Cook Time: 2.5 Minutes
Yields: 2 tbsps

Ingredients:

2 shallots, peeled and thinly sliced
2 tbsps olive oil

Directions:

1. Put the sliced shallots in a small microwave bowl. Almost cover with the oil.
2. Microwave for approximately 2.5 minutes, checking progress after first minute then every 30 seconds. Remove shallots when they are just brown as they continue cooking in the hot oil.
3. When shallots turn golden brown, drain and let cool.
4. Store in an air tight container to keep cool.

Nutritional Information per serving:

Calories: 64
Fat: 7g
Carbs: .8g
Dietary fibre: 0g
Protein: .1g
Cholesterol: 0mg
Sodium: 1mg

SOUPS

SCOTCH BROTH

Total Time: 2 Hours 15 Minutes
Prep Time: 35 Minutes
Cook Time: 1 Hour 40 Minutes
Yields: 4 servings

Ingredients:

2.2lbs/1kg lamb neck chops
3/4 cup pearl barley
9 cups (2.25 litres) water
1 1/2 tbsps onion flakes or other onion substitute
2 medium carrots (½ lb/240g) cut into ½ inch (1cm) pieces
1 medium leek (14oz/350g) leek, sliced thinly
2 cups (5.5oz/160g) finely shredded cabbage
1/2 cup coarsely chopped flat leaf parsley

Directions:

1. Place the lamb, barley and the water in a large saucepan and bring to the boil over medium heat. Reduce heat and simmer, covered for 1 hour. Skim off any fat that rises to the surface.
2. Add the carrot, onion, and leek, and simmer, covered, until the carrot is tender, approx. 30 minutes.
3. Remove the lamb from pan and let cool in order to remove the bones. Shred the lamb coarsely and place it back in the soup, discarding the bones.
4. Add the cabbage to the soup and simmer uncovered for 10 minutes, or until cabbage is just tender.

5. Sprinkle the parsley over the soup when serving.

Nutritional Information per serving: (Serving size: 1 cup):

Calories: 594
Fat: 22.7g
Carbs: 38.9g
Dietary fibre: 8.1g
Protein: 55.8g
Cholesterol: 166mg
Sodium: 229mg

CAULIFLOWER AND BROCCOLI SOUP

Prep Time: 10 Minutes
Cook Time: 20 Minutes
Yields: 4 servings

Ingredients:

1 cauliflower, cut into florets
1 head broccoli, including stem, coarsely chopped
1 tbsp. olive oil
1 tsp ground cumin
2 tsp sweet paprika
2 garlic cloves, crushed
1 1/2 tbsps onion flakes or other onion substitute
2 sweet potatoes, peeled, coarsely chopped
4 cups chicken stock
1/2 cup coconut cream or other dairy milk substitute

Directions:

1. Heat oil in a large heavy bottomed saucepan over medium-high heat. Add garlic and onion substitute (if using) and cook for 5 minutes. Add cumin and paprika and cook, stirring for 1 minute or until fragrant. Add a splash of stock to combine spices.
2. Add broccoli, cauliflower, sweet potato, onion flakes (if using), and chicken stock to the pot and bring to the boil. Reduce heat to medium-low and simmer, partially covered, for approximately 20 minutes. Vegetables should be soft, but not overcooked. Broccoli should still be bright green.

3. Transfer mixture to a blender in batches and blend until smooth, or use a stick blender in the pan. Stir in the coconut cream, and season with salt and pepper.

Nutritional Information per serving: (Serving size: 1 cup):

Calories: 255
Fat: 11.9g
Carbs: 12.9g
Dietary fibre: 8.6g
Protein: 6.6g
Cholesterol: 0mg
Sodium: 871mg

CARROT AND GINGER SOUP

Total Time: 35 Minutes
Prep Time: 10 Minutes
Cook Time: 25 Minutes
Yields: 4 servings

Ingredients:

1 tbsp. butter substitute such as coconut oil
2.2lbs/1kg small carrots, peeled, diced
1.5 inch (4cm) piece fresh ginger, peeled, grated
2 cups vegetable stock
1 cup water
1/2 cup coconut cream or other dairy milk substitute
3 tsps chopped fresh tarragon
salt & ground black pepper

Directions:

1. In a large saucepan over medium heat melt the butter substitute. Add the carrots and ginger and stir to coat. Cover and cook, until the carrots have softened, approx. 10 minutes, stirring occasionally with a wooden spoon. Add the water and stock and bring to the boil. Simmer, uncovered, approx. 10 minutes, until the carrots are tender.
2. Blend the soup in batches in a blender until smooth. Alternatively use a stick blender in the pan.
3. Return the soup to the pan and heat over medium heat, adding the coconut cream and tarragon. Heat through, stirring, for approx. 3 minutes. Season with salt and pepper.

Nutritional Information per serving: (Serving size: 1 cup), based on the above ingredients. Information will vary if other substitutes are used.

Calories: 220
Fat: 12.6g
Carbs: 26.6g
Dietary fibre: 6.9g
Protein: 2.9g
Cholesterol: 0mg
Sodium: 179mg

CHICKEN NOODLE SOUP

Total Time: 45 Minutes
Prep Time: 20 Minutes
Cook Time: 25 Minutes
Yields: 4 servings

Ingredients:

1lb (400g) chicken breast fillet, poached
1 packet thin Hokkien noodles
1 teaspoon dried chilli
4 cups chicken stock
6 cups water
2 tbsps onion flakes or other onion substitute
2 garlic cloves, crushed

Directions:

1. Prepare Hokkien noodles according to the directions on the packet.
2. Poach chicken: place enough water in a saucepan to cover the chicken and set to boil. Reduce heat to simmer and add the chicken, poaching for 15 minutes or until chicken is cooked through.
Drain and let chicken cool before shredding it.
3. In a large stock pot heat the oil over a medium heat, add the garlic and cook for one minute.
Add the carrots and celery and cook until soft, approximately 5 minutes.
4. Add the stock and water and bring to the boil. Add the salt, pepper, rosemary, dried chilli and onion flakes.

5. Add the chicken and parsley and reduce heat to medium low. Simmer uncovered for 15 - 20 minutes.
6. Add noodles and simmer for another five minutes. Season with salt and pepper if desired.

Nutritional Information per serving: (Serving size: 1 cup):

Calories: 250
Fat: 9.4g
Carbs: 6.4g
Dietary fibre: 1g
Protein: 30.6g
Cholesterol: 89mg
Sodium: 952mg

SWEET POTATO AND PUMPKIN SOUP

Total Time: 35 Minutes
Prep Time: 10 Minutes
Cook Time: 25 Minutes
Yields: 4 servings

Ingredients:

2 tbsp olive oil
1.1lb (500g) sweet potato, peeled, roughly chopped
2.2lb (1kg) butternut pumpkin roughly chopped
1 tbsp fresh ginger finely grated
1½ tbsps onion flakes or other onion substitute
1 tbsp ground cumin
4 cups vegetable stock
1/2 cup water

Topping:

1/3 cup chopped fresh coriander
1 long fresh red chilli, deseeded, finely chopped
2 tbsps shredded coconut
Coconut cream, to serve

Directions:

1. In a large saucepan heat the oil over medium low. Cook half the ginger, stirring, for 2 minutes. Add the pumpkin, sweet potato, and half the cumin. Cook, stirring, for 2 minutes or until fragrant.

2. Add the water and stock, increase heat to high and bring to the boil. Reduce heat and simmer for 15 minutes. Pumpkin and sweet potato should be very tender. Stand for 5 minutes to cool slightly. Transfer to a blender and process until smooth. Season with salt and pepper.
3. In a small bowl combine the chilli, coriander, coconut and remaining ginger.
4. Divide the soup among serving bowls and top with the coconut mixture.

Nutritional Information per serving: (Serving size: 1 cup):

Calories: 305
Fat: 9.3g
Carbs: 49.6g
Dietary fibre: 12.2g
Protein: 6g
Cholesterol: 0
Sodium: 62mg

CHICKEN, VEGETABLE AND PASTA SOUP

Total Time: 1 Hour
Prep Time: 10 Minutes
Cook Time: 50 Minutes
Yields: 1.5 litres

Ingredients:

2 chicken breast fillets
1 sweet potato, diced
2 medium carrots, diced
1/2 cup chopped broccoli
2 celery sticks, diced
2 cloves garlic, finely diced
8 cups chicken or vegetable stock
1 medium zucchini, diced
1½ tbsps onion flakes or other onion substitute
1 tbsp. olive oil
pepper
1 cup small pasta or risoni

Directions:

1. Poach chicken: place enough water in a saucepan that will cover the chicken and set to boil. Reduce heat to simmer and add the chicken, poaching for 15 minutes or until chicken is cooked through. Drain and allow chicken to cool before shredding it.
2. In a large saucepan heat the oil over a medium heat and cook the garlic, stirring. Add the vegetables and stir until softened, approximately 5 minutes.

3. Add the stock and pasta and bring to the boil. Reduce heat and simmer, partially covered, stirring occasionally until pasta is cooked, approximately 20 minutes. Add extra stock if needed.
4. Add the chicken and pepper, and simmer for another 5 minutes.

Nutritional Information per serving: (Serving size: 1 cup):

Calories: 465
Fat: 12.5g
Carbs: 19.8
Dietary fibre: 2.7g
Protein: 64.5g
Cholesterol: 175g
Sodium: 173mg

APPETISERS / SIDES

COCONUT RICE

Total Time: 35 Minutes
Prep Time: 5 Minutes
Cook Time: 30 Minutes
Yields: 6 servings

Ingredients:

3 cups jasmine rice, well-rinsed
1.5 inch (3cm) piece ginger, peeled, halved
13.5 oz. (400ml) can coconut cream
3 cups cold water

Directions:

1. Combine all ingredients in a large pan and bring to a boil, stirring occasionally.
2. Reduce heat to a simmer. Cook for 10 minutes, covered.
3. Take off heat and stand for 10 minutes, covered. Remove ginger. Serve.

Nutritional Information per serving:
Calories: 626
Fat: 14g
Carbs: 117g
Dietary fibre: 4.2g
Protein: 7g
Cholesterol: 34mg
Sodium: 88mg

PARSNIP PUREE

Total Time: 60 Minutes
Prep Time: 15 Minutes
Cook Time: 45 Minutes
Yields: 10 servings

Ingredients:

10 medium parsnips (4 lbs/1.8kg), peeled and chopped into
1/2-inch-thick slices
3/4 cup (170g) butter substitute such as coconut oil
1/2 cup chicken stock
1 tbsp fine sea salt
2 teaspoons freshly ground black pepper

Directions:

1. Place parsnips in a large saucepan and cover with cold water. Cover and bring to the boil over moderately high heat.
2. Continue to boil until tender, approximately 30 to 45 minutes. Drain.
3. Puree the parsnips in batches with the butter/coconut oil and chicken stock. Stir in salt and pepper.

Nutritional Information per serving:

Calories: 248
Fat: 17.4g
Carbs: 24g
Dietary fibre: 6.5g
Protein: 1.6g
Cholesterol: 0mg
Sodium: 613mg

CAULIFLOWER WITH CUMIN AND TURMERIC

Total Time: 18 Minutes
Prep Time: 10 Minutes
Cook Time: 8 Minutes
Yields: 4 servings

Ingredients:
1½lbs (700g) cauliflower, cut into small florets
1 teaspoon cumin seeds
1 inch (2cm) piece fresh ginger, finely grated
1 tsp ground turmeric
1/3 cup coconut cream
2 tbsps roughly chopped fresh coriander leaves

Directions:
1. In a large bowl combine the cauliflower, cumin, ginger, and turmeric. Add salt and pepper if desired. Mix to coat.
2. Bring a large saucepan of water to the boil and place the cauliflower mixture in a covered metal steamer over the top. Reduce the heat to low and simmer, steaming the cauliflower for 8 minutes.
3. Place in a large serving bowl. Add coconut cream and coriander and gently combine. Serve hot.

Nutritional Information per serving:
Calories: 102
Fat: 5.3g /
Carbs: 12.7g /
Dietary fibre: 5.3g
Protein: 4.3g
Cholesterol: 0mg
Sodium: 57mg

POLENTA FRITTERS

Total Time: 23 Minutes
Prep Time: 15 Minutes
Cook Time: 8 Minutes
Yields: 8 Servings

Ingredients:

2 tsps olive oil
salt
1¼ cups (220g) polenta (cornmeal)
1 cup vegetable stock
1 egg
7oz (200ml) water
¼ cup (60ml) hot water

Directions:

1. Whisk the stock and egg together in a medium saucepan. Add the water and stir.
2. Turn on heat to medium and gradually add the polenta, in a continuous stream, until all combined with the liquid. Season with salt and stir continuously for 3-4 minutes, or until mixture is bubbling. Continue cooking for a further 2-3 minutes, stirring occasionally, until mixture thickens. Take the saucepan off the heat, and stir in the hot water.
3. In a large non-stick frying pan heat the oil over medium-high heat. Use approximately 1/3 cup of the mixture for each fritter (about 4 inches / 10cm in diameter). Flatten with an egg lifter if desired. Cook for 2-3 minutes each side, turning carefully. Remove from pan and keep warm on a plate by covering with foil.

Nutritional Information per serving: (Serving size: 1/2 cup):

Calories: 237
Fat: 3.9g
Carbs: 44.2g
Dietary fibre: 1.2g
Protein: 5.6g
Cholesterol: 41mg
Sodium: 56mg

ZUCCHINI AND CORN FRITTERS

Total Time: 20 Minutes
Prep Time: 5 Minutes
Cook Time: 15 Minutes
Yields: 4 servings

Ingredients:
6 oz. (150g) zucchini, grated
Medium size (310g) tin corn kernels, drained
2 tbsps olive oil
2 eggs, lightly beaten
1/3 cup coconut milk or other dairy milk substitute
1 cup self-raising flour
1/2 tsp ground cumin
salt and pepper

Directions:
1. Place the zucchini, corn, eggs and milk in a bowl and whisk together.
2. In another bowl mix together the flour, cumin, and salt and pepper.
3. Slowly stir the flour mix into the wet mix.
4. In a frying pan heat the olive oil over medium heat. Using heaped tbsps, cook in batches, ensuring to cook through.

Nutritional Information per serving:
Calories: 321
Fat: 15.1g
Carbs: 41.1g
Dietary fibre: 3.2g /
Protein: 9g
Cholesterol: 82mg
Sodium: 270mg

CAULIFLOWER PUREE

Prep Time: 10 Minutes
Cook Time: 20 Minutes
Yields: 4 Servings

Ingredients:

1 head (small) (2.2 lb/1kg) white cauliflower, cut into small florets
2 tbsps (30g) coconut oil or other butter substitute

Directions:

1. Cook cauliflower in a large saucepan of boiling water for 15 to 20 minutes, until it is very tender. Thoroughly drain in a colander and return to saucepan.
2. Add butter substitute and mash until it reaches your desired consistency. Season with salt and cracked black pepper. Serve.

Nutritional Information per serving:

Calories: 117
Fat: 7.7g
Carbs: 11.1g
Dietary fibre: 5.2g
Protein: 4.3g
Cholesterol: 0mg
Sodium: 63mg

PEARL BARLEY AND PUMPKIN RISOTTO

Total Time: 45 Minutes
Prep Time: 10 Minutes
Cook Time: 35 Minutes
Yields: 4 servings

Ingredients:

1¾ lb (800g) pumpkin, chopped into 1.5cm pieces
3 cups chicken stock
2 tsps olive oil
olive oil in pump spray
2 cloves garlic, smashed
1½ tbsps onion flakes or other onion substitute
1 cup (220g) pearl barley - soak overnight and drain
2/3 cup (160ml) white wine substitute: Verjus / white grape juice / apple juice
1 bunch rocket, coarsely chopped
2 tsps fresh rosemary, chopped

Directions:

1. Preheat oven to 350ºF/180ºC. Line a baking tray and place the pumpkin on it. Spray with oil and bake until just cooked, approx. 25 minutes.
2. In a large saucepan heat oil on medium heat. Add garlic and stir for one minute. Mix in the rosemary and barley.
3. Add verjus/juice and onion flakes to barley mix. Reduce mixture by half by simmering.

4. At the same time, heat the stock until it boils, then reduce to a simmer. Add 1/2 cup to the reduced barley mix. Cook over medium heat, stirring continuously until the liquid absorbs. Continue adding stock, approximately 1/2 cup each time, ensuring the liquid is nearly all absorbed before stirring in another 1/2 cup. Continue until the barley becomes tender, approx. 20 to 25 minutes.
5. Add the cooked pumpkin and rocket. Cover and stand 5 minutes before serving.

Nutritional Information per serving:

Calories: 324
Fat: 4.1g
Carbs: 68g
Dietary fibre: 4.8 g
Protein: 8.5g
Cholesterol: 0mg
Sodium: 624mg

SWEET POTATO, ZUCCHINI AND RICOTTA SLICE

Total Time: 55 Minutes
Prep Time: 15 Minutes
Cook Time: 40 Minutes
Yields: 4 servings

Ingredients:

2 teaspoons olive oil
10.5oz (300g) sweet potato, peeled, roughly grated
1 1/2 tbsps onion flakes or other onion substitute
2 cloves garlic, smashed
4 eggs
2 egg whites
1/2 cup fresh ricotta (reduced-fat)
1/2 lb (250g) zucchini, grated, and fluid removed*
1/4 cup (40g) plain (all purpose) flour
2 tbsps fresh chives, chopped
2 tbsps fresh continental parsley, chopped
10in x 6in (26cm x 16cm) slice pan

Directions:

1. Preheat oven to 350ºF/180ºC. Grease and line the slice pan.
2. In a large frying pan heat oil over high. Cook the sweet potato for approximately 4 minutes, until soft. Add the garlic and stir for 1 minute.
3. In a large bowl whisk the flour, 4 eggs and 2 egg whites until smooth. Gently stir in ricotta, then the zucchini, sweet potato mix, parsley and chives.

4. Pour mixture into prepared slice pan. Bake 25 to 30 minutes, testing the centre with a skewer to ensure cooked through. Cool slightly before serving.

*Remove moisture from zucchini by wringing it with your hands, or putting in a sieve and pressing it with the back of a spoon.

Nutritional Information per serving:

Calories: 215
Fat: 7.1g
Carbs: 27.8g
Dietary fibre: 3.7g
Protein: 11g
Cholesterol: 164mg
Sodium: 123mg

SPINACH, PUMPKIN AND RICOTTA PENNE

Total Time: 27 Minutes
Prep Time: 15 Minutes
Cook Time: 12 Minutes
Yields: 4 servings

Ingredients:

3/4 lb (350g) penne pasta
2 cloves garlic, smashed
3/4 lb (350g) butternut pumpkin, chopped into1 inch (2cm) cubes
1/2 teaspoon chilli flakes
1 tbsp olive oil
olive oil in pump spray
1 tbsp reconstituted onion flakes or other onion substitute
1/2 cup (120g) ricotta cheese (reduced-fat)
5oz. (150g) baby spinach

Directions:

1. Preheat oven to 350ºF/180ºC. Cook pasta according to packet directions in a large saucepan.
2. Arrange pumpkin on a lined baking tray and spray with olive oil. Bake until just cooked, approximately 25 minutes.
3. In a large frying pan heat oil over medium heat. Cook garlic, other onion substitute if using, for 3 minutes. Add chilli and pumpkin and cook 2 minutes.

4. Drain the pasta and return to saucepan. Stir in pumpkin mixture, onion flakes (if using), spinach and ricotta. Heat through over low heat for a few minutes until spinach has just wilted. Season with salt and pepper and serve.

Nutritional Information per serving:

Calories: 367
Fat: 8.2g
Carbs: 59.4g
Dietary fibre: 3.5g
Protein: 15.1g
Cholesterol: 71mg
Sodium: 102mg

ANGEL HAIR PASTA WITH SALMON RICOTTA

Total Time: 25 Minutes
Prep Time: 10 Minutes
Cook Time: 15 Minutes
Yields: 4 servings

Ingredients:
1 lb (500g) angel hair pasta
3 tbsp olive oil
10oz (300g) fresh salmon
9 oz (250g) ricotta
5oz (150g) baby spinach
Salt and black pepper

Directions:
1. Cook pasta according to the directions on the packet.
2. Heat oil on low heat in a medium saucepan. Add the salmon, using a fork to mash slightly.
3. Cook for 2 minutes until salmon and olive oil have mixed together.
4. Reduce heat to low and stir through ricotta.
5. When the pasta has cooked, drain and add immediately to the pan.
6. Mix baby spinach through and season with salt and cracked pepper and serve immediately.

Nutritional Information per serving:
Calories: 644
Fat: 23.1g
Carbs: 73g
Dietary fibre: 0.8g
Protein: 36.9g
Cholesterol: 144mg
Sodium: 173mg

FETTUCINI WITH CREAMY PUMPKIN SAUCE

Total Time: 27 Minutes
Prep Time: 15 Minutes
Cook Time: 25 Minutes
Yields: 4 Servings

Ingredients:

1 lb (500g) fettuccine
1½ lb (750g) pumpkin, peeled and chopped into small pieces
1½ cups vegetable stock
1 cup coconut cream or full fat yogurt
1½ tbsps onion flakes or other onion substitute
1 clove garlic, chopped
2 tbsp (30g) butter substitute such as coconut oil
Nutmeg
Pepper to taste

Directions:

1. Cook pasta as directed on the packet and drain.
2. In a large saucepan over medium heat, melt the butter substitute and cook onion substitute (if using) and garlic. Stir until soft and fragrant.
3. Stir in vegetable stock, pumpkin and onion flakes (if using). Cook until pumpkin is tender.
4. Add nutmeg and pepper and stir in coconut cream/yogurt.
5. In batches, transfer mixture to blender and process until smooth.
6. Stir the sauce through pasta. Serve immediately.

Nutritional Information per serving:

Calories: 307
Fat: 6.4g
Carbs: 87.1g
Dietary fibre: 6.8g
Protein: 17.6g
Cholesterol: 91mg
Sodium: 51mg

MAINS

PORK

PORK CUTLETS WITH PARNSIP MASH

Prep Time: 10 Minutes
Cook Time: 30 Minutes
Yields: 4 servings

Ingredients:

5 parsnips, peeled, sliced
2 2/3 cups (660ml) coconut milk
3 garlic cloves – 2 whole, 1 finely chopped
2 tbsps olive oil
4 pork cutlets
3½ tbsps (50g) butter substitute such as coconut oil
3 green apples, peeled, cut into 1cm-thick wedges
2 teaspoons caster sugar
1/4 cup sage leaves

Directions:

Parsnip Mash:
1. In a saucepan heat the coconut milk, parsnips, and 2 whole garlic cloves to just below boiling point, then reduce heat to medium-low. Simmer until parsnips are tender, approximately for 15 minutes. Take the garlic and the parsnips from the milk and keep the milk.

2. In a food processer, place the finely chopped garlic clove, the cooked whole garlic, the cooked parsnip, and 1/2 cup milk. Blend until smooth. Add more milk if needed. Season with salt and pepper.

Port Cutlets:
Season the cutlets with salt and pepper. In a frying pan over medium high, heat 1 tbsp oil. Cook the cutlets for 2-3 minutes each side until just cooked through. Remove from pan and rest, covered loosely with foil.

Apple:
1. In the same frying pan, heat butter substitute and remaining tbsp oil. Cook the apple, caster sugar, seasoning, for 5 minutes, until the apple is tender and has a light caramelisation. Mix in sage leaves for 1 minute until wilted.
2. To serve, plate up the parsnip mash, topped by the pork, then the apple. Drizzle with pan juices.

Nutritional Information per serving:

Calories: 773
Fat: 57.9g
Carbs: 73.5
Dietary fibre: 13.7g
Protein: 16.4g
Cholesterol: 50mg
Sodium: 1664g

HERB CRUMBED PORK WITH CAULIFLOWER PUREE

Prep Time: 15 Minutes
Cook Time: 25 Minutes
Yields: 4 Servings

Ingredients:

4 pork cutlets
1/4 cup (40g) plain (all purpose) flour
1 cup (90g) breadcrumb substitute: cornflake breadcrumbs
or homemade day old breadcrumbs
2 tsp s ground fennel
2 tbsps chopped fresh continental parsley
2 eggs, lightly whisked in a small bowl
1/2 cup (125ml) olive oil

Cauliflower Puree:
1 small head (2.2lb/1kg) white cauliflower, cut into small
florets
2 tbsps (30g) coconut oil or other butter substitute

Directions:

1. Bring a large saucepan of water to the boil over high
   heat. Add cauliflower. Cook for 15 to 20 minutes or until
   cauliflower is very tender.
2. While the cauliflower is cooking, pound pork until 1 inch
   (2cm) thick using the flat side of a meat mallet.
3. Place the flour on a large plate. Mix together the
   breadcrumbs, parsley and fennel, and place on another
   plate.

4. Lightly dust pork in flour, dunk in egg and evenly coat in breadcrumbs. Place on a tray.
5. In a frying pan heat olive oil over medium high. Fry the cutlets for 2 to 3 minutes on both sides until golden and cooked through.
6. Drain the cauliflower and return to saucepan. Add butter substitute and mash until almost smooth. If a smoother texture is desired, blend in a blender. Season with salt and cracked black pepper.

Nutritional Information per serving:

Calories: 577
Fat: 42g
Carbs: 21g
Dietary fibre: 6.2g
Protein: 17.3g
Cholesterol: 30mg
Sodium: 563mg

STEAK WITH COCONUT CREAM SPINACH

Prep Time: 15 Minutes
Cook Time: 25 Minutes
Yields: 4 Servings

Ingredients:

3½ lb (1.5kg) orange sweet potato, peeled, cut into 7mm-thick rounds
4 pork loin medallion steaks
5 oz. (150ml) coconut cream
2 bunches trimmed and washed English spinach
1 small finely chopped fresh red chilli
1 finely chopped garlic clove
1½ tbsp. olive oil

Directions:

Preheat the oven to 400°F/200°C.
1. Coat sweet potato with tbsp oil and bake until tender, for about 25 minutes.
2. In the meantime, add one teaspoon oil to a frying pan and heat over medium-high. Add pork and cook until cooked through, about 3-4 minutes each side. Transfer to a plate, cover with a foil and let stand.
3. Heat the rest of the oil in the same frying pan over medium-high; add chilli and garlic and sauté until fragrant, for about 30 seconds. Stir in spinach and coconut cream for about 2 minutes or until spinach starts to wilt.

4. Divide the cooked sweet potato among serving plates and top with spinach mixture and pork. Serve immediately.

Nutritional Information per serving:

Calories: 782
Fat: 25.6g
Carbs: 86.2g
Dietary fibre: 17.1 g
Protein: 58g
Cholesterol: 0mg
Sodium: 1275mg

ASIAN SPICED PORK RISSOLES

Total Time: 35 Minutes
Prep Time: 20 Minutes
Cook Time: 15 Minutes
Yields: 4-6 servings

Ingredients:

2 cups steamed jasmine rice
2 Lebanese cucumbers
1 lightly beaten egg
1½ lb (750g) pork mince
1/2 cup coriander leaves
4 roughly chopped green onions
1 stalk lemongrass, bruised
2 small roughly chopped red chillies
1½ inch (3cm) piece peeled and grated fresh ginger
2 chopped garlic cloves
olive oil

Directions:

1. Combine coriander, green onions, lemongrass, chilli, garlic and ginger in a food processor and pulse until finely chopped. Transfer the mixture to a bowl; add the egg, pork mince, salt and pepper and mix to combine well.
2. Form 16 balls from the mixture, flattening slightly. Arrange the balls on a plate and refrigerate, covered, for at least 30 minutes.

3. Heat a large frying pan over medium-low heat. Add oil to the pan and cook the rissoles, turning occasionally, until cooked through, for about 15 minutes.
4. Serve the rissoles with jasmine rice and cucumber slices.

Nutritional Information per serving:

Calories: 606
Fat: 6.7g
Carbs: 132.7g
Dietary fibre: 3.1g
Protein: 6.4g
Cholesterol: 27mg
Sodium: 44mg

PORK CUTLETS WITH BEAN MASH

Total Time: 30 Minutes
Prep Time: 15 Minutes
Cook Time: 15 Minutes
Yields: 4 servings

Ingredients:

1 3/4 lb (800g) fresh or equivalent after soaking dried cannellini beans or 2 x 13.5 oz (400g) cans rinsed and drained
1 cup chicken stock
1 tbsp. butter substitute such as coconut oil or olive oil spread
1/4 cup cranberry sauce
4 trimmed pork cutlets
2 tsp. olive oil
1 tbsp. finely chopped rosemary leaves
Steamed broccolini, to serve

Directions:

1. Evenly season both sides of pork with salt and pepper. In a heavy-based frying pan, heat oil over medium heat. Add pork and cook for about 5 minutes per side. Transfer the cooked pork to a plate and cover with foil; set aside.
2. Add ¼ cup stock and cranberry sauce to pan and cook over medium heat, stirring constantly, until smooth. Add the remaining stock and bring the mixture to a boil; cook until reduced by half, for about 2 minutes.

3. In the meantime, blend rosemary and cannellini beans in a blender or food processor until almost smooth. Transfer the mixture to a saucepan; add butter substitute and stir over medium heat until heated through, for about 5 minutes. Add salt and pepper and cover until ready to serve.
4. To serve, divide bean mixture between two serving plates; top each with a pork cutlet, drizzled with the sauce. Serve the bean mash with steamed broccolini.

Nutritional Information per serving:

Calories: 371
Fat: 9.4g
Carbs: 32.4g
Dietary fibre: 15.3g
Protein: 37.2g
Cholesterol: 83mg
Sodium: 582mg

CHICKEN AND TURKEY

TURKEY AND CRANBERRY SCHNITZELS

Total Time: 45 Minutes
Prep Time: 20 Minutes
Cook Time: 25 Minutes
Yields: 8 servings

Ingredients:

Cranberry jelly
Olive oil for frying
4 (about 3 lbs. / 1.3kg) turkey breast fillets
4 cups breadcrumbs substitute such as cornflake crumbs or homemade day old
3 lightly beaten eggs
1/3 cup plain (all purpose) flour
3/4 cup cranberry sauce

Directions:

Preheat the oven to 350ºF/180ºC fan-forced. Line a baking dish with baking paper and set aside.

1. Slice turkey into 1/2 inch (1 cm)-thick slices or in half horizontally, pressing gently to flatten. Evenly spread one side of each slice of turkey with the cranberry sauce, and then lightly dust with flour. Dip the turkey slices in the egg before coating evenly with breadcrumbs. Arrange the slices onto a tray.

2. Add oil, up to 1/2 inch (1 cm high), to a large non-stick frying pan and set over medium heat. Working in batches, add the coated turkey slices, starting with cranberry side down, and cook until cooked through and golden, for about 2-3 minutes per side.
3. Transfer to the prepared baking tray and bake until just cooked through, for about 8 minutes. Drain on paper towel before serving.

Nutritional Information per serving:

Calories: 427
Fat: 17g
Carbs: 29.4g
Dietary fibre: 2g
Protein: 19.1g
Cholesterol: 78mg
Sodium: 306mg

CHICKEN AND SPINACH BAKE

Total Time: 50 Minutes
Prep Time: 25 Minutes
Cook Time: 35 Minutes
Yields: 4 Servings

Ingredients:

2 oz. (50g) cornflake crumbs or other breadcrumb substitute
5 oz. (150g) baby spinach
1½ tbsp. cornflour
2 cups coconut milk or other dairy milk substitute
1/2 cup chicken stock
1 tbsp. fresh sage, chopped
10½ oz (300g) peeled and grated butternut pumpkin
1.1 lb (500g) chicken mince
1½ tbsp. onion flakes or other onion substitute
1 tbsp. olive oil
1/2 lb (250g) penne pasta

Directions:

Preheat the oven to 400°F/200°C. Follow package instructions to cook pasta; drain and keep warm.

1. In the meantime, set a large frying pan with oil over medium high heat; sauté onions (if using), stirring occasionally, until tender, for about 5 minutes. Add chicken mince and cook until browned, for about 10 minutes.
2. Add coconut milk, onion flakes (if using), stock, sage and pumpkin; simmer, uncovered, for about 5 minutes or until pumpkin is just tender.

3. In a bowl, mix together 2 tbsp. water and cornflour until well combined; stir the mixture into the sauce and continue cooking, stirring continuously, for about 2 minutes or until the sauce boils and becomes thick. Mix in pasta and spinach and season with salt and pepper if desired.
4. Transfer the mixture to a standard 12-cup ovenproof baking dish; sprinkle with cornflake crumbs and bake for about 15 minutes.

Nutritional Information per serving: (Serving size: 1 cup), based on the above ingredients. Information will vary if using other substitutes.

Calories: 718 /
Fat: 19.4g /
Carbs: 14g /
Dietary fibre: 6.2g /
Protein: 34g /
Cholesterol: 153mg /
Sodium: 239mg

CHICKEN AND VEGETABLE FRICASSE

Total Time: 50 Minutes
Prep Time: 15 Minutes
Cook Time: 35 Minutes
Yields: 6 servings

Ingredients:

Cooked risoni
1½ lb (750g) trimmed and quartered chicken thigh fillets
1½ tbsp. olive oil
2 finely chopped garlic cloves
2 tbsp. plain (all purpose) flour
1/3 cup white wine substitute such as apple juice/white grape juice/Verjus
1½ cups chicken stock
2 tbsp. fresh tarragon leaves, chopped
1/4 cup coconut cream
2 cups fresh vegetables
1 1/2 tsp. dried tarragon leaves

Directions:

1. Heat two teaspoons oil in a non-stick frying pan over medium high. Sprinkle chicken thigh fillets with salt and pepper and add to the frying pan, in batches; cooking until golden, about 3 minutes per side. Transfer chicken to a plate and set aside.
2. Add the remaining oil to pan and heat. Stir in garlic until fragrant, for about 1 minute. Stir in flour for 2 minutes.

3. Remove the frying pan from heat; stir in juice/wine until the mixture is smooth. Stir in dried tarragon and stock. Return the pan to heat and cook, stirring constantly, until the mixture thickens, for about 6 minutes.
4. Return chicken to the frying pan and continue cooking, stirring frequently, until cooked through, about 12 minutes.
5. In the meantime, blanch vegetables in boiling water for about 10 seconds and drain.
6. Add the vegetables and cream to the chicken mixture and cook until warmed through, about 3 minutes.
7. Add fresh tarragon, salt and pepper; stir to mix well. Serve with risoni.

Nutritional Information per serving:

Calories: 409
Fat: 18.9g
Carbs: 31.1g
Dietary fibre: 2g
Protein: 28.2g
Cholesterol: 0mg
Sodium: 208mg

CRANBERRY TURKEY MEATLOAF

Total Time: 26 Minutes
Prep Time: 25 Minutes
Cook Time: 1 Minute
Yields: 8 servings

Ingredients:

1/2 cup melted cranberry jelly
3/4 cup cornflake crumbs or other breadcrumbs substitute
1 lightly beaten egg
2.2lb (1kg) turkey mince
1/4 cup fresh sage leaves, shredded
2 crushed garlic cloves
1 grated green apple
½ tbsp. reconstituted onion flakes or other onion substitute
2 tbsp. fresh flat-leaf parsley leaves, chopped

Directions:

Preheat the oven to 350°F/180°C (fan-forced). Prepare a 5.5 x 4.5 inch (14×12 cm), 2½ inch (6cm)-deep loaf pan by greasing and lining with baking paper.

1. In a bowl, combine together apple, onion flakes/substitute, egg, turkey, breadcrumbs, parsley, sage and garlic. Mix with your hands until well blended. Press the mixture into the prepared loaf pan.
2. In a saucepan, gently melt the cranberry jelly over medium heat. Brush meatloaf top with two tbsps melted cranberry jelly. Bake until cooked through, for about 1 hour. Let the meatloaf cool in the pan for at least 5 minutes before lifting it from pan with a paper lining.

3. Place the meatloaf onto a plate and brush with the remaining cranberry juice before serving.

Nutritional Information per serving, based on the above ingredients. Information will vary if other substitutes are used:

Calories: 202
Fat: 7.7g
Carbs: 7.8g
Dietary fibre: 1.5g
Protein: 26g
Cholesterol: 20mg
Sodium: 27mg

INDIAN CHICKEN AND CAULIFLOWER PILAF

Total Time: 26 Minutes
Prep Time: 10 Minutes
Cook Time: 20 Minutes
Yields: 4 servings

Ingredients:

3/4 lb (350g) chicken breast fillets, diced
1 cup frozen peas
3/4 lb (350g) cauliflower, cut into small florets
1½ cups basmati rice
2 tbsp. olive oil
2¼ cups chicken stock
1/2 cup chopped fresh coriander leaves
1 small deseeded and finely chopped red chilli
1 tsp. ground turmeric
1½ tbsp. onion flakes or other onion substitute
Coconut cream to serve

Directions:

1. Heat oil in a large saucepan over medium high. Add chicken and cook for about 2-3 minutes or until browned. Transfer the chicken to a plate.

2. Lower the heat to medium and sauté onion substitute if using, in the pan until tender, for about 3minutes. Add rice, chilli, turmeric, and continue cooking, stirring, until fragrant, for about 30 seconds. If using onion flakes add now, then cauliflower, chicken, and stock. Raise heat to high and bring the mixture to a gentle boil. Lower heat to medium-low, cover and cook until rice is almost tender, for about 10 minutes.
3. Add peas, cover and cook until stock has been absorbed and rice is tender, about 3 minutes. Remove the pan from heat and let stand, covered, for at least 5 minutes.
4. Add half the coriander and stir to combine well.
5. To serve, top with the remaining coriander and a dollop of coconut cream.

Nutritional Information per serving, based on the above ingredients. Information will vary if other substitutes are used.

Calories: 545
Fat: 14.6g
Carbs: 67.8g
Dietary fibre: 5.3g
Protein: 34.6g
Cholesterol: 78mg
Sodium: 538mg

GINGER CHICKEN MEATBALLS

Total Time: 17 Minutes
Prep Time: 10 Minutes
Cook Time: 7 Minutes
Yields: 4 Servings

Ingredients:

2 tbsp. olive oil
14 oz (400g) chicken mince
1 cup bread crumb substitute such as cornflake or day old homemade
1 cup medium-grain white rice, cooked
1 lightly beaten egg
1 deseeded and finely chopped birds eye chilli
2 crushed garlic cloves
1½ inch (3cm) piece finely grated fresh ginger
2 thinly sliced green onions
1/2 cup fresh coriander leaves, finely chopped
Coriander leaves, to serve

Directions:

1. In a large bowl, combine together ginger, onion, coriander, garlic, breadcrumbs, rice, egg, chicken mince, chilli, salt and pepper. Using your hands, mix the ingredients until well combined.
2. Form small balls from the mixture using level tbsps and place them on a plate.

3. Heat oil in a large frying pan over medium high. Add the meatballs and cook, turning frequently, for about 7 minutes or until cooked through and browned on the surface.

Nutritional Information per serving:

Calories: 259
Fat: 9.5g
Carbs: 44.1g
Dietary fibre: 1.4g
Protein: 3.7g
Cholesterol: 0mg
Sodium: 199mg

AYAM GORENG WITH COCONUT RICE

Total Time: 4 Hours 30 Minutes
Prep Time: 3 Hours 25 Minutes
Cook Time: 1 Hour 5 Minutes
Yields: 6 Servings

Ingredients:

2 tsps olive oil
12 mixed chicken pieces
13.5 oz. (400ml) can coconut milk
1 tsp. ground turmeric
2 tsp. sea salt
2 tsp. ground coriander
1 stick chopped lemongrass (white part only)
3/4 inch (2cm) piece fresh ginger, peeled, chopped
1½ tbsp. reconstituted onion flakes, or other onion substitute
olive oil, for frying

Coconut rice:
2 cups water
2 cups jasmine rice
3/4 inch (2cm) piece peeled and halved fresh ginger
13.5 oz. (400ml) can coconut milk

Directions:

1. Rinse the chicken pieces and pat dry with paper towel. Refrigerate, uncovered, to dry out well.
2. In a food processor, blend together coriander, lemongrass, ginger, onion, 1/4 cup coconut milk, turmeric and salt until finely chopped.

3. Heat oil over medium high in a frying pan. Add the coconut mixture from the processor and cook, stirring constantly, until fragrant, for about 1 minute. Add the chicken pieces, skin side down. Pour the remaining coconut milk over the chicken and bring to a boil. Lower the heat to low and simmer for about 15 minutes, uncovered. Turn the chicken and cook the other sides for another 15 minutes.

4. Transfer the chicken mixture to a plate and place in the refrigerator, uncovered, for at least 3 hours and up to 12 hours if possible.

5. Make coconut rice: combine together all the ingredients in a large saucepan and bring to a boil, stirring occasionally. Lower heat to low, cover and simmer until liquid is absorbed, for about 10 minutes. Discard ginger.

6. Finish cooking chicken: add enough oil to a deep frying pan and heat over medium high. Working in batches, cook chicken pieces until golden, for about 3 minutes per side; drain with paper towels on a large plate and serve with the cooked coconut rice, garnished with coriander.

Nutritional Information per serving, based on the above ingredients. Information will vary if other substitutes are used.

Calories: 939
Fat: 39.5
Carbs: 56.6g
Dietary fibre: 4.2
Protein: 50g
Cholesterol: 130mg
Sodium: 842mg

CHICKEN LEGS WITH TURMERIC RICE

Total Time: 70 Minutes
Prep Time: 15 Minutes
Cook Time: 55 Minutes
Yields: 4 Servings

Ingredients:

2 cups basmati rice
8 chicken legs
4 cups chicken stock
1 tbsp. olive oil
1 tsp. ground chilli powder
2 tsp. ground turmeric
1 tbsp. ground coriander
1 tbsp. grated ginger
2 garlic cloves, crushed
1/2 cup chopped coriander

Directions:

1. Preheat the oven to 350°F/180°C. Heat a tbsp of olive oil in a medium frying pan over medium heat. Add chicken legs and cook, turning frequently, until cooked through; transfer to a plate and set aside.
2. Add rice, chilli powder, turmeric, ground coriander, ginger and garlic to the pan and stir until well blended. Transfer the mixture to an 8-cup ovenproof baking dish and top with the chicken legs. Pour chicken stock over the mixture and bake for about 40 minutes.

3. Remove the chicken legs and stir in ½ cup coriander until well blended. Serve the chicken legs and turmeric rice with coconut cream.

Nutritional Information per serving:

Calories: 655
Fat: 15.3g
Carbs: 77g
Dietary fibre: 1.7g
Protein: 48.2g
Cholesterol: 125mg
Sodium: 934mg

CHICKEN TAGINE WITH SWEET POTATO AND GINGER

Total Time: 65 Minutes
Prep Time: 20 Minutes
Cook Time: 45 Minutes
Yields: 4 Servings

Ingredients:

1.3 lb (600g) chicken thigh fillets, trimmed, halved
2 cups chicken stock
1 medium peeled carrot, sliced
1/2 lb (250g) chopped sweet potato
1 tbsp. olive oil
1½ tbsp. onion flakes or other onion substitute
1/2 tsp. ground cinnamon
1 tsp. ground coriander
1 tsp. ground cumin
1.5 inch (4cm) piece peeled and grated fresh ginger
2 chopped garlic cloves
1/2 cup chopped fresh coriander leaves

Directions:

Preheat oven to 350°F/180°C.
1. In a large heavy-based casserole dish heat half the oil over medium heat. Working in batches, cook chicken until it is browned, for about 4 minutes each side. Transfer chicken to a plate.

2. Heat the remaining oil and cook the onion substitute if using, stirring until tender, for about 5 minutes. Add cinnamon, coriander, cumin, ginger and garlic and cook until fragrant, for about 1 minute.
3. Stir in carrot and sweet potato until well coated. Add onion flakes if using, stock and chicken; bake, covered, until chicken is cooked and vegetables are tender, for about 30 minutes.
4. Stir in coriander and honey and season with pepper to serve.

Nutritional Information per serving:

Calories: 343
Fat: 16g
Carbs: 15.9g
Dietary fibre: 2.5g
Protein: 35g
Cholesterol: 143mg
Sodium: 549mg

SEAFOOD

MARINATED SWORDFISH WITH CANNELLINI BEANS

Total Time: 33 Minutes
Prep Time: 15 Minutes
Cook Time: 18 Minutes
Yields: 4 Servings

Ingredients:

2/3 cup chicken stock
1 3/4 lb. (800g) fresh or equivalent after soaking, dried cannellini beans or 2 x 14oz (400g) cans rinsed and drained
2 shallots, finely chopped
4 x 1/2 lb (200g) swordfish steaks
1/4 cup olive oil
2 tbsp. fresh oregano leaves
6 garlic cloves - 2 sliced and 4 finely chopped.
2 tbsp. flat-leaf parsley, and more to garnish, roughly chopped
2 rosemary sprigs

Directions:

1. In a dish, mix together garlic, oregano, and two tbsps oil. Season fish with salt and pepper, and then coat in the garlic mixture and let marinate while you prepare the beans.

2. Heat one tbsp oil in a large frying pan over medium low. Add shallots and chopped garlic and cook, stirring constantly, until starting to colour, for about 6 minutes. Increase heat to medium, add rosemary, stock and cannellini beans; simmer the mixture until stock is almost absorbed, for about 5 minutes. Discard rosemary sprigs.

3. Place one cup of the bean mixture into a bowl and coarsely mash with a wooden fork. Return the mashed mixture to the pan and stir for 1 more minute. Add parsley and stir to mix well; keep warm.

4. Set a chargrill or a frying pan over high heat. Add swordfish and sear until cooked to your liking, about 2 minutes per side.

5. Divide the bean mixture among four serving plates; top each with swordfish and sprinkle with more parsley. Serve immediately.

Nutritional Information per serving:

Calories: 344
Fat: 17.4g
Carbs: 33.1g
Dietary fibre: 11.1g
Protein: 65g
Cholesterol: 40mg
Sodium: 228g

CRISPY SKIN SALMON TWO WAYS

Total Time: 30 Minutes
Prep Time: 5 Minutes
Cook Time: 10 Minutes
Yields: 4 Servings

Ingredients:

4 (about 1/2 lb/200g each) salmon fillets, with skin
1 tsp. sea salt
2 tbsp. olive oil

Method 1 Directions:

1. Arrange fish, skin side up, on a large plate; sprinkle with oil and rub salt into the skin.
2. Heat a large non-stick frying pan on medium high. Add the salmon, skin side down and cook for about 5 minutes, until skin is crisp. Turn the fish, cover pan and continue cooking until fish is cooked, about 5 minutes, or to your liking.

Method 2 Directions:

Preheat oven to 350°/180°C.
1. Place salmon, skin side up, on a plate. Coat with oil and rub salt into skin.

2. Heat an oven-proof frying pan on medium-high heat. Wait until the pan is hot before adding the salmon, skin side down. The skin should start to crisp in 1 minute of cooking. Turn it and cook for 30 seconds, then put the pan in the oven and bake for 5 minutes, or until cooked, but still a little rare in the centre.

Nutritional Information per serving:

Calories: 300
Fat: 13g
Carbs: 0g
Dietary fibre: 0g
Protein: 39g
Cholesterol: 88mg
Sodium: 88mg

COCONUT CRUMBED CHILLI FISH

Total Time: 30 Minutes
Prep Time: 15 Minutes
Cook Time: 15 Minutes
Yields: 4 Servings

Ingredients:

1 tbsp. olive oil
1 1/3 cups shredded coconut
6 (4 oz/120g each) boneless or flathead white fillets, cut into halves lengthwise
1 lightly beaten egg
2 tbsp. coconut milk
1/2 tsp. dried chilli flakes
Asian greens and steamed jasmine rice, to serve

Directions:

1. Combine together coconut and chilli flakes on a plate. In a bowl, beat together the egg and milk. Prepare a baking tray by lining it with baking paper and set aside.
2. Dip the fillets into the milk mixture, then into the coconut mixture. Arrange them on the prepared baking tray.
3. Heat oil in a large frying pan over medium heat. Add fish and cook until cooked through, for about 3 minutes per side.

Serve fish with Asian greens and steamed jasmine rice.

Nutritional Information per serving:

Calories: 142
Fat: 14.2g
Carbs: 4.5g
Dietary fibre: 6g
Protein: 1.1g
Cholesterol: 0mg
Sodium: 6mg

SPINACH WRAPPED FISH PARCELS

Total Time: 22 Minutes
Prep Time: 10 Minutes
Cook Time: 12 Minutes
Yields: 2 Servings

Ingredients:

4 x 6.5 oz. (180g) boneless white fish fillet
4 large silverbeet leaves, with no stems
Olive oil cooking spray
3.5 inch (4cm) piece fresh ginger, peeled, sliced
1 garlic clove, thinly sliced
Salt
Ground pepper
Noodles or steamed rice, to serve

Directions:

1. Set a non-stick frying pan over medium high heat.
2. Coat 4 foil sheets with olive oil. Place silverbeet leaf in the centre of each sheet. Place the fish on the leaf and sprinkle with ginger, garlic, salt and pepper.
3. Fold silver beet leaf over the fish fillet and seal the ends to form a parcel. Place the parcels into the frying pan and cook for about 6 minutes per side.
4. Drizzle with any juices from the parcels, coconut aminos (soy sauce substitute). Serve with noodles or rice.

Nutritional Information per serving:

Calories: 250
Fat: 3g
Carbs: 2g
Dietary fibre: 2g
Protein: 29g
Cholesterol: 97mg
Sodium: 230mg

FISH IN COCONUT MILK

Total Time: 40 Minutes
Prep Time: 20 Minutes
Cook Time: 20 Minutes
Yields: 4 Servings

Ingredients:

1 3/4 lb (800g) firm white fish fillets, cubed
13.5oz (400ml) can coconut milk
10 fresh curry leaves
2 garlic cloves, crushed
1 long deseeded and finely chopped green chilli
1 tsp. turmeric
1 tsp. ground coriander
1½ tbsp. onion flakes or other onion substitute
1 tbsp. olive oil
Steamed basmati rice and pappadums
Coriander leaves

Directions:

1. Heat oil in a large frying pan over medium. Add curry leaves, garlic, chilli, coriander, and turmeric; cook, stirring constantly, for about 1 minute or until fragrant.
2. Add coconut milk, lower heat to medium low and let the mixture simmer until slightly reduced, for about 10 minutes. Add fish and continue cooking until fish is just cooked through, for about 5 minutes.
3. Add seasoning and top with coriander leaves. Serve the fish with pappadums and basmati rice.

Nutritional Information per serving:

Calories: 618
Fat: 42.8g
Carbs: 8.1g
Dietary fibre: 2.5g
Protein: 51.6g
Cholesterol: 154mg
Sodium: 146mg

COCONUT PRAWNS

Total Time: 30 Minutes
Prep Time: 10 Minutes
Cook Time: 20Minutes
Yields: 4 Servings

Ingredients:

13.5 oz. (400ml) can coconut milk
24 medium green prawns
1 tsp. curry powder
1 small red chilli, finely chopped
1 tsp. ginger, finely grated
1 chopped garlic clove
1½ tbsp. reconstituted onion flakes or other onion substitute
2 tsp. olive oil
Steamed rice, to serve
Fresh basil leaves, torn

Directions:

1. Add a cup of water to a saucepan and bring to a boil. Lower heat, add prawns and simmer, covered, until prawns are cooked through, for about 5 minutes. Transfer to a bowl to cool.
2. When cool, remove prawns from water, reserving water. Peel and devein the cooked prawns and return the shells to the reserved water.
3. Heat oil in a small saucepan over medium heat. Add ginger, chilli, garlic and curry powder; cook, stirring, until fragrant and golden, for about 2 minutes.

4. Add reserved water to the pan with spices, discarding prawn shells. Add onion flakes and coconut milk and bring the mixture to a boil. Lower heat to low and let the mixture simmer for at least 10 minutes. Stir in prawns and basil until just heated and serve with rice.

Nutritional Information per serving:

Calories: 258
Fat: 26.6g
Carbs: 6.5g
Dietary fibre: 2.5g
Protein: 2.5g
Cholesterol: 0mg
Sodium: 16mg

CRISPY CAULIFLOWER AND FISH BAKE

Total Time: 55 Minutes
Prep Time: 20 Minutes
Cook Time: 35 Minutes
Yields: 4 Servings

Ingredients:

4 slices wholemeal bread (day old), torn into large chunks
1.3 lb (600g) cauliflower, sliced
1 tbsp. chopped dill
14 oz (400g) pink ling fish fillets, cubed
2 tbsp. olive oil
2½ cups coconut milk or other dairy milk substitute
1 clove garlic, finely chopped
1 celery stick, diced
2 small carrots, diced
1½ tbsp. reconstituted onion flakes or other onion substitute
Salt & pepper

Directions:

Preheat the oven to 425°F/220°C fan forced.

1. Combine milk and cauliflower in a medium saucepan and bring to a gentle simmer over medium heat until cauliflower is tender, about 7 minutes.
2. Strain the cooked cauliflower, reserving milk.
3. Transfer cauliflower to a food processor and pulse until thick and smooth. Add the reserved milk, if necessary and season with salt and pepper; set aside.

4. Heat one tbsp oil in a frying pan over medium heat. Add garlic, carrots and celery and cook until tender, for about 5 minutes. Season with salt and pepper. Add dill, reconstituted onion flakes, cauliflower puree and fish; mix until well combined. Transfer to coated baking dish.
5. In a bowl, toss together one tbsp oil and bread; pour over the fish mixture and bake until bread is golden brown, for about 20 minutes.

Nutritional Information per serving:

Calories: 367
Fat: 7.9
Carbs: 26.2g
Dietary fibre: 7.8g
Protein: 44.4g
Cholesterol: 77mg
Sodium: 465mg

MEAT

LAMB AND BARLEY IRISH STEW

Total Time: 1 Hour 30 Minutes
Prep Time: 20 Minutes
Cook Time: 1 Hour 10 Minutes
Yields: 4 Servings

Ingredients:

1 bunch trimmed and shredded English spinach
2 cups chicken stock
4 (1.75 lb/760g) lamb forequarter chops, with bones
1 cup pearl barley
1½ tbsp. onion flakes or other onion substitute
3 tbsp. plain (all purpose) flour
1 tbsp. olive oil
2 carrots, halved lengthways and thickly sliced
1 large celery stalk, trimmed, thickly sliced
1 tsp. dried thyme
Salt and pepper

Directions:

1. Trim the lamb of fat and pat dry. Toss the lamb in seasoned flour until well coated.
2. Heat oil in a heavy-based saucepan over medium high heat. Add lamb, in batches, and cook until browned, for about 4 minutes.

3. Add ½ cup cold water, onion flakes/substitute, thyme, stock, barley, salt and pepper and bring to a boil, covered. Lower heat to low and simmer the mixture until barley is almost tender, for about 40 minutes.
4. Add carrot and celery and continue simmering until barley and lamb is tender, for about 20 minutes.
5. Remove the pan from heat and stir in spinach until wilted.
6. Remove bones from lamb and serve.

Nutritional Information per serving, based on above ingredients. Will vary if other substitutes are used:

Calories: 447
Fat: 15.6g
Carbs: 51.5g
Dietary fibre: 11g
Protein: 28.3g
Cholesterol: 60mg
Sodium: 542mg

CRANBERRY LAMB SHANKS WITH CREAMED SPINACH

Total Time: 2 Hours 50 Minutes
Prep Time: 5 Minutes
Cook Time: 2 Hours 45 Minutes
Yields: 4 Servings

Ingredients:

1/4 cup low-fat coconut cream
4 lamb shanks (about 4½ lb/2kgs)
2 bunches English spinach, trimmed, leaves washed and dried
20g butter substitute such as coconut oil or olive oil spread
4 garlic cloves, finely chopped
2 tbsp. fresh rosemary leaves
2 tbsp. wholegrain mustard
1/2 cup red wine substitute such as cranberry juice
1 x small (275g) jar cranberry sauce
Salt and ground black pepper

Directions:

Preheat the oven to 300°F/150°C.
1. Season the lamb shanks with salt and pepper and place them in a roasting pan.
2. In a bowl, combine together two garlic cloves, rosemary, mustard, juice, and cranberry sauce. Pour the mixture over the lamb, cover with foil and bake for about 2½ hours, turning occasionally, until tender. Remove pan from oven and raise temperature to 430°F/220°C.

3. Drain the pan juices into a saucepan. Return the lamb shanks to oven and bake, uncovered, until browned, for about 15 minutes, turning once during cooking time.
4. In the meantime, set the saucepan with juices over high and bring to a boil. Cook, stirring occasionally, until sauce thickens, for about 8 minutes.
5. Melt butter substitute in a large frying pan over high heat. Stir in the remaining garlic until fragrant, for about 30 seconds. Add spinach and stir until just wilted, about 2 minutes. Stir in cream and bring the mixture to a boil. Season with salt and pepper if desired.
6. To serve, divide spinach among serving plates, top with lamb and drizzle with sauce.

Nutritional Information per serving:

Calories: 240
Fat: 9.7g
Carbs: 33g
Dietary fibre: 5.4g
Protein: 33g
Cholesterol: 450mg
Sodium: 238mg

ROAST LAMB RACK WITH ROSEMARY AND MUSTARD CRUST

Total Time: 40 Minutes
Prep Time: 10 Minutes
Cook Time: 30 Minutes
Yields: 8 Servings

Ingredients:

2 trimmed and quartered zucchini
4 French trimmed lamb racks
8 yellow squash, halved
1 tbsp. fresh rosemary, chopped
2 tbsp. wholegrain mustard
Olive oil spray
1.6 lb (750g) peeled and cubed Kent pumpkin

Directions:

Preheat the oven to 390°F/200°C.
1. Line a large baking dish with non-stick baking paper. Brush the pumpkin with oil and transfer to the prepared baking dish. Season the pumpkin with pepper and bake until tender, for about 15 minutes.
2. In the meantime, set a large frying pan coated with oil over high heat. Add the lamb racks and cook for about 2 minutes or until browned.
3. In a bowl combine together mustard and rosemary and spread 1/4 of the mixture over each lamb rack.

4. When pumpkin is done, add zucchini and squash to the baking dish, top with the lamb racks and bake for about 15 minutes or until the lamb is cooked to your liking. Transfer the lamb to a plate, cover with a foil and let cool for at least 5 minutes. Continue cooking until the vegetables are tender.

Nutritional Information per serving:

Calories: 378
Fat: 12.8g
Carbs: 16.1g
Dietary fibre: 5.6g
Protein: 49.9g
Cholesterol: 154mg
Sodium: 1387 mg

SLOW COOKER MADRAS BEEF CURRY

Total Time: 5 Hours 15 Minutes
Prep Time: 15 Minutes
Cook Time: 5 Hours
Yields: 6 servings

Ingredients:

3/4 cup chicken stock
9 fl.oz (270ml) light coconut milk
1/4 cup plain (all purpose) flour
1/4 cup Indian madras curry paste
1 long red chilli, chopped finely
1.5 inch (4cm) piece peeled and grated fresh ginger
2 crushed garlic cloves
14oz (400g) sweet potatoes
1½ tbsp. onion flakes or other onion substitute
2 tbsp. olive oil
1lb12oz (800g) diced beef
1 bay leaf
1 cinnamon stick
low-fat coconut cream, steamed rice, and chopped fresh coriander, to serve

Directions:

1. Mix together flour, beef, salt and pepper in a plastic bag and shake gently to coat the beef. Cook beef in a saucepan in batches on medium high heat until browned, about 4 minutes. Place the browned beef in a slow cooker.

2. In the same saucepan, cook the ginger and garlic (and other onion substitute if using), for about 5 minutes. Add curry paste and chilli and cook until fragrant, for about 1 minute. Add stock, onion flakes (if using), and coconut milk; bring the mixture to a boil. Add the mixture with beef to the slow cooker. Stir in bay leaf and cinnamon stick until well combined.

3. Cover and cook on low until beef is tender, for about 6 hours. Remove from heat, discarding bay leaf and cinnamon. Serve the curry with low-fat coconut cream, rice, day old naan bread and coriander.

Nutritional Information per serving:

Calories: 496
Fat: 24.1g
Carbs: 26.4g
Dietary fibre: 4g
Protein: 43.3g
Cholesterol: 119mg
Sodium: 116mg

SWEDISH MEATBALLS

Total Time: 50 Minutes
Prep Time: 15 Minutes
Cook Time: 35 Minutes
Yields: 4 Servings

Ingredients:

1/2 cup coconut cream
1 tsp. cornflour
3/4 cup beef stock
1/4 cup olive oil
1 egg lightly beaten
1/8 tsp. ground allspice
1 garlic clove, crushed
I tbsp. reconstituted onion flakes or other onion substitute
1.1lb (500g) beef mince
1/4 cup coconut cream, extra
1/2 cup breadcrumb substitute such as day old, homemade
freshly ground pepper
1/2 tsp. salt

Directions:

1. Add coconut cream to a large bowl and soak the breadcrumbs. Add beef mince, egg, allspice, garlic, reconstituted onion flakes, salt and pepper; mix to combine well. Form small meatballs from the mixture.

2. Heat oil in a large frying pan over medium high. Add the meatballs, in batches, and cook until brown. Drain off any excess oil and return the meatballs to the pan. Add stock, and simmer, covered, for about 20 minutes. Transfer the meatballs to a plate and keep warm.
3. In a bowl, mix together cornflour and water; stir into the meatball mixture to thicken. Bring the mixture to a boil; lower heat to low, add extra coconut cream and cook for about 1 minute, stirring.
4. Pour the sauce over the meatballs and serve.

Nutritional Information per serving:

Calories: 504
Fat: 32g
Carbs: 13g
Dietary fibre: 1.7g
Protein: 41.4g
Cholesterol: 625mg
Sodium: 679mg

BEEF AND PUMPKIN CURRY

Total Time: 25 Minutes
Prep Time: 5 Minutes
Cook Time: 20 Minutes
Yields: 6 Servings

Ingredients:

1-2 tbsp. red curry paste
2 tbsp. olive oil
1.1lb (500g) beef (rump), sliced thinly
14oz (400g) peeled and cubed butternut pumpkin
2 tsp brown sugar
1/2 cup beef stock
1 cup coconut cream
1/2 cup fresh basil leaves
Optional: 2 tbsp. Thai fried shallots

Directions:

Combine the beef and 1 tbsp. of the oil in a bowl. Heat a large frying pan over medium-high and stir-fry one third of the beef until seared, about 2 minutes. Transfer to a bowl. Reheat the pan and repeat in 2 batches.
Clean the pan and heat until just hot. Add the remaining oil and curry paste and stir until fragrant. Add the pumpkin, sugar, stock, and cream and stir until well combined. Simmer until pumpkin is just soft, for about 8 minutes.
Add the cooked beef, cover, and simmer gently for another 2 minutes.
To serve, scatter with fried shallots and chopped basil leaves before serving with rice.

Nutritional Information per serving:

Calories: 170
Fat: 15.2
Carbs: 9.1g
Dietary fibre: 2.8g
Protein: 1.9g
Cholesterol: 205mg
Sodium: 261mg

DESSERTS

GINGER GOLDEN SYRUP PUDDING

Total Time: 50 Minutes
Prep Time: 20 Minutes
Cook Time: 30 Minutes
Yields: 8 servings

Ingredients:

1/2 cup golden syrup
1/3 cup milk
1/2 teaspoon ground cinnamon
1/2 teaspoon baking powder, sifted
1 1/2 cups self-raising flour, sifted
2 eggs
2/3 cup caster sugar
5oz (150g) butter substitute, such as coconut oil
2 inch (5cm) piece fresh ginger, peeled

Directions:

1. Prepare a 6-cup pudding basin by coating lightly with oil, and cutting a circle from the baking paper, with a lid as a guide.
2. Finely grate 1cm ginger slice and slice the remaining into matchsticks.
3. With an electric beater, cream the sugar and butter substitute until fluffy and light. Beat in the eggs, one at a time, until well combined. Stir in the finely grated ginger. Stir in cinnamon, flour, baking powder, and half the milk.

4. Combine sliced ginger and golden syrup in a large bowl; spoon into the bottom of the pudding dish then add the batter. Smooth the surface, cover the basin with baking paper and secure with a lid.

5. Place an inverted saucer in a large saucepan and sit the basin on top. Add boiling water to the saucepan until half full. Cover and bring to a simmer over medium heat, then lower heat to medium low and simmer, adding boiling water as necessary, for about 2 hours. Test with a skewer.

6. Carefully remove the pudding basin from the saucepan. Let stand for 5 minutes before turning onto a plate. Serve with extra golden syrup and coconut cream.

Nutritional Information per serving:

Calories: 312
Fat: 16.2g
Carbs: 41g
Dietary fibre: 0.6g
Protein: 3.3g
Cholesterol: 33mg
Sodium: 42mg

COCONUT WHIPPED CREAM

Total Time: 10 Minutes
Prep Time: 10 Minutes
Cook Time: 0 Minutes
Yields: 500grams

Ingredients:

Vanilla
Sugar
13.5 oz (400g) can full-fat coconut milk

Directions:

1. Chill a can of coconut milk for at least 8 hours, or overnight. When chilled, scoop out the solidified top layer of the milk, stopping when you reach the liquid.
2. Transfer the coconut cream to a large bowl and beat with an electric mixer on high for about 5 minutes or until light and fluffy with soft peaks. Stir in vanilla sugar if desired.

Nutritional Information per 20g serving:

Calories: 25
Fat: 2.4g
Carbs: 0.8g
Dietary fibre: 0.5g
Protein: .2g
Cholesterol: 0mg
Sodium: 7mg

BAKED RICE PUDDING

Total Time: 25 Minutes
Prep Time: 10 Minutes
Cook Time: 15 Minutes
Yields: 4 Servings

Ingredients:

2 egg yolks
2 tsp. vanilla bean paste
10 fl.oz (300ml) low-fat coconut cream
2 cups coconut milk or other dairy milk substitute
1 cinnamon stick
1/3 cup caster sugar
1/2 cup rinsed and drained Arborio or calrose rice
Pinch ground nutmeg

Directions:

Preheat the oven to 320°F/160°C.
1. In a medium saucepan set over medium heat, combine together sugar, rice, coconut cream, coconut milk, vanilla and cinnamon. Cook, stirring occasionally, for about 5 minutes or until the mixture comes to a gentle simmer. Remove the pan from the heat and let stand for at least 15 minutes for flavours to infuse. Discard cinnamon.
2. Stir in egg yolks until well combined.
3. Transfer the mixture into a 4-cup ovenproof baking dish; sprinkle with nutmeg and bake, stirring occasionally, until custard is set and rice is tender, for about 1 hour. Remove pudding from oven and cool for at least 10 minutes before serving.

Nutritional Information per serving based on the above ingredients. Information will vary when other substitutes are used:

Calories: 300
Fat: 20.7g
Carbs: 28.1g
Dietary fibre: 2g
Protein: 3.8g
Cholesterol: 70mg
Sodium: 15mg

CORNBREAD WITH BLUEBERRIES

Total Time: 40 Minutes
Prep Time: 10 Minutes
Cook Time: 30 Minutes
Yields: 6 servings

Ingredients:

5 oz (150g) blueberries
3 tbsp (60g) butter substitute, such as coconut oil, melted and cooled
1 cup coconut milk or other dairy milk substitute
2 eggs
1 cup corn meal
1 cup plain (all-purpose) flour
1/4 cup caster sugar
3 teaspoons baking powder
4 x 8.5 x 2.5 inch (10cm x 22cm x 6cm) loaf tin

Directions:

Preheat the oven to 350°F/180°C. Lightly coat the loaf tin with cooking spray and line with baking paper.
1. In a large bowl, sift together flour, baking powder and corn meal. Add the caster sugar and stir until well combined. Make a hollow in the centre of the mixture.
2. In a separate bowl, whisk together eggs, melted butter substitute and coconut milk. Gradually add to the dry mixture in the formed hollow, stirring in circles until all ingredients are only just combined - do not over mix. Fold in the blueberries.

3. Spoon the batter into the lined baking tin and bake for about 40 minutes, testing with a skewer to ensure it is cooked. Remove bread from oven and let cool in the tin for at least 5 minutes before transferring to a wire rack to cool completely. Great served with butter and honey.

Nutritional Information per serving:

Calories: 403
Fat: 22g
Carbs: 49.3g
Dietary fibre: 4.1g
Protein: 7.2g
Cholesterol: 73mg
Sodium: 29mg

PEACH GINGERBREAD COBBLER

Total Time: 50 Minutes
Prep Time: 20 Minutes
Cook Time: 30 Minutes
Yields: 4 servings

Ingredients:

2 cups plain (all-purpose) flour
1/2 cup brown sugar
1 egg
2 tbsps butter substitute, melted
1/4 cup golden syrup
1/2 cup coconut milk or other dairy milk substitute
28oz (815g) can peach halves in natural juice
1/4 tsp. ground nutmeg
1/2 tsp. ground ginger
1/2 tsp. bicarbonate of soda
1/2 tsp. baking powder
Whipped coconut cream, to serve

Directions:

Preheat the oven to 390°F/200°C.
1. Drain the peach pieces, reserving 1/4 cup juice.
2. Arrange the peaches cut side up, in a shallow 5-cup baking dish. Pour the reserved juice over the peaches.
3. Using a large bowl, whisk together egg, butter substitute, syrup, coconut milk, and sugar until well blended.

4. Sift together flour, nutmeg, ginger, bicarbonate of soda, and baking powder. With a large metal spoon, fold the dry ingredients into the wet mixture to make the batter - do not over mix.
5. Top the peaches with batter, leaving some small gaps, and bake for about 30 minutes or until a tester inserted in the centre comes out clean. Serve the gingerbread cobbler warm with coconut cream.

Nutritional Information per serving based on the above ingredient. Information will vary if other substitutes are used:

Calories: 404
Fat: 12.9g
Carbs: 68.4g
Dietary fibre: 3.6g
Protein: 6.9g
Cholesterol: 27mg
Sodium: 39mg

CRANBERRY POACHED PEARS

Total Time: 35 Minutes
Prep Time: 10 Minutes
Cook Time: 25 Minutes
Yields: 4 Servings

Ingredients:

4 ripe pears, peeled, halved and cored
1 cinnamon stick
1/4 cup brown sugar
4 cups cranberry juice

Directions:

1. Combine brown sugar and cranberry juice in a medium sized saucepan and cook, stirring, over medium heat until sugar is dissolved. Add pears and cinnamon and bring the mixture to a boil.
2. Lower heat to low, partially cover the saucepan, and simmer until pears are tender, for about 15 minutes. Discard cinnamon.
3. Transfer pears to a plate and set aside, keeping warm.
4. Strain about 1½ cups of the liquid from the saucepan into a tall jug, discarding the rest. Return the reserved liquid to the pan and bring to a gentle boil. Let cook until the liquid becomes a syrup and reduced by half, about 10 minutes.
5. Drizzle the pears with the syrup and top with a dollop of coconut whipped cream or coconut cream. Serve immediately.

Amanda Kent

Nutritional Information per serving:

Calories: 191
Fat: 2g
Carbs: 52.8g
Dietary fibre: 10.8g
Protein: 1.1g
Cholesterol: 0mg
 Sodium: 7mg

GINGERNUT BISCUITS

Total Time: 50 Minutes
Prep Time: 30 Minutes
Cook Time: 20 Minutes
Yields: 30

Ingredients:

1 tbsp. boiling water
1 tsp. bicarbonate of soda
1 tsp. ground cinnamon
3 tsp. ground ginger
1 cup golden syrup
3 cups plain (all-purpose) flour, sifted
1 cup, firmly packed soft brown sugar
9oz (250g) butter substitute, such as coconut oil

Directions:

Preheat the oven to 350°F/180°C. Prepare two baking trays by lining them with non-stick baking paper.
1. Combine golden syrup, brown sugar, butter substitute, cinnamon and ginger in a large saucepan over medium heat; stir to blend well. Continue cooking the mixture, stirring often, until almost boiling.
2. Transfer the mixture to a large bowl and let cool for about 10 minutes.
3. Combine water and bicarbonate of soda; stir until bicarbonate of soda is completely dissolved. Add to the wet mixture and stir. Stir in flour until well blended.

4. With a teaspoon, spoon the batter onto the prepared baking trays, forming 3cm rounds, leaving enough room for each round to spread.
5. Bake until golden brown, for about 10 minutes. Remove the biscuits from oven and let cool on baking trays. Repeat the procedure until all the mixture is finished.

Store the biscuits in airtight container.

Nutritional Information per serving: (Serving size: 1 x 3.5oz/100g cookie), based on the above ingredients. Information will vary if other substitutes are used.

Calories: 77
Fat: 2.9g
Carbs: 13.4g
 Dietary fibre: 1.1g
Protein: 1.3g
Cholesterol: 0mg
Sodium: 112mg

ANZAC BISCUITS

Total Time: 1 Hour 10 Minutes
Prep Time: 55 Minutes
Cook Time: 15 Minutes
Yields: 24 Servings

Ingredients:

1/2 cup butter substitute such as coconut oil
3/4 cup caster sugar
1 cup desiccated coconut
1 cup plain (all-purpose) flour
1 cup rolled oats
1 tbsp. boiling water
1 tsp. bicarbonate of soda
2 tbsp. golden syrup

Directions:

1. Preheat your oven to 350°F/180°C fan-forced. Prepare two baking trays by lining them with baking paper.
2. Sift all-purpose flour into a large bowl. Stir in sugar, coconut and oats until well combed. Make a well in the middle of the mixture.
3. Heat golden syrup and butter in a saucepan over medium heat, stirring, until butter substitute is melted.
4. Stir bicarbonate of soda into one tbsp of boiling water until completely dissolved; stir into the butter mixture until well blended.
5. Add the butter mixture to the flour mixture and stir until well blended.

6. Using level tbsps, form balls from the mixture and arrange them, 1.5 inch (3 cm) apart, on the lined baking trays, flattening slightly. Bake, swapping the baking trays halfway during cooking time, until golden, for about 15 minutes. Let cool on the baking trays for at least 5 minutes before transferring to a wire rack to completely cool.

Nutritional Information per serving: (Serving size: 1 cookie) based on the above ingredients. Information will vary if other substitutes are used.

Calories: 100
Fat: 4.9g
Carbs: 13g
Dietary fibre: 0g
Protein: 1.3g
Cholesterol: 0mg
Sodium: 70mg

COMMON INGREDIENT SUBSTITUTES

BUTTER:
- Coconut Oil 1:1 - Coconut Oil has a lower melting point than butter, so for recipes where the butter has to be hard, such as creaming butter with sugar, measure the amount you need and put it in the freezer until it's really cold. It's also a good idea to put the bowl and utensils you are going to use in the refrigerator or freezer as well. Note that coconut oil is much higher in calories than butter.
- Olive oil spread
- Vegetable shortening can be used for crusts and pastry 1:1 - Tip: Use a pastry cutter that has been placed in the freezer along with the other utensils when cutting the pastry.

DAIRY MILK:
- Coconut Milk 1:1
- Other milks such as Soy or Rice.

YOGHURT:
- Coconut Cream - but be aware it has a higher fat content
- For hearty dishes – medium firm silken tofu.

ONION:
- Onion flakes
- Shallots
- Leeks
- Green onions (spring onions)

How to use onion flakes:
Add onion flakes directly to the dish if it contains adequate liquid. If it is a dry dish, reconstitute first by soaking in cold water for half an hour. Use 1 /4 cup of onion flakes for each fresh onion called for in your recipe, or the following guide:
- 1/2 tbsp for small
- 1 tbsp for medium
- 1½ tbsp for a large one

VINEGAR:
White rice vinegar is okay in small amounts. All other vinegars are triggers.

YEAST:
Avoid fresh baked bread products. However, after 24 hours the yeast is not a trigger. It's the fresh-baked yeast products that will give you trouble due to the tyramine they contain.

SESAME OIL:
Cold-pressed/expellar-pressed, <u>not toasted</u>.

PACKAGED BREADCRUMBS:
- Cornflake crumbs
- Homemade breadcrumbs from day old bread can be safely used.

RED WINE:
Juices such as: grape, pomegranate, cranberry, pink grapefruit

WHITE WINE:
- Verjus
- White grape juice
- Apple juice

BREAD:
Any type of freshly baked bread can be a trigger because of the freshly risen yeast. Packaged bread doesn't present this problem, but it may contain preservatives which can also be a migraine trigger, so check the packaging. A good idea is to buy freshly baked and leave it overnight, by which time it is safe to eat.

SOY SAUCE:
Coconut Aminos 1:1

Amanda Kent

Also by the author of the Migraine Diet Cookbook

Migraine Diet Smoothies

Every recipe completely migraine trigger FREE!

Over 30 delicious and healthy smoothies WITHOUT migraine triggers.
All smoothies include ingredients that contain nutrients beneficial for migraine sufferers.

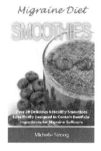

OTHER BOOKS BY SCG PUBLISHING

Keto Make Ahead Freezer Meals & Snacks by Skye Howard RDLD
Keto Smoothies and Shakes by Skye Howard RDLD
Keto One Pot Meals by Skye Howard RDLD

HIIT: High Intensity Interval Training - Look Like An Athlete, Feel Like An Athlete by Steve Ryan MScExerciseand NutritionBScSport

Printed in Great Britain
by Amazon